Embracing the Sounds of Change:

A Journey Through Hearing Loss and the Power of Hearing Aids

Dedication

To all the brave souls who embark on the journey toward better hearing, this book is dedicated to you. May you find the strength, resilience, and inspiration within these pages to embrace your transformation and discover the beautiful symphony of life that awaits you. Remember, you are not alone; let the harmony of support guide you as you navigate the path to improved hearing and a life filled with connection and joy.

Table of Contents

Dedication 2

Introduction.. 7

Chapter 1: The Silent Garden - Acknowledging Your Hearing Loss 8

The journey to rediscovering your world of sound begins by acknowledging the change that has occurred in your life. Like a once-vibrant garden that has grown silent and still, it's essential to recognize the beauty that remains and embrace the possibility of renewal.

    1.1 The Beauty in Silence 8

    1.2 The Fading Notes 9

    1.3 The Seeds of Change 9

    1.4 Cultivating Self-Compassion 9

    1.5 The Power of Vulnerability 10

    1.6 Turning the Soil.. 10

Chapter 2: The Echo of Self-Acceptance - Embracing Your Reality... 11

Accepting your hearing loss as part of your reality is a crucial step toward positive change. Discover the power of self-acceptance, as it echoes through your life and creates a foundation for self-improvement and growth.

2.1 The Sound of Acceptance 11

2.2 The Layers of Self-Acceptance 11

2.3 The Mirror of Self-Reflection 12

2.4 The Warmth of Self-Compassion 12

2.5 The Strength of Vulnerability 12

2.6 The Ripple Effect of Acceptance 13

Chapter 3: The Whispering Wind - Listening to Your Inner Voice 14

Your inner voice can be your most significant source of guidance and motivation. Learn to listen to the whispers of your intuition and trust your ability to make decisions that will lead you toward a better quality of life.

3.1 The Gentle Breeze of Intuition 14

3.2 Clearing the Mental Clutter 14

3.3 Trusting Your Inner Guidance 15

3.4 Overcoming Self-Doubt 15

3.5 The Power of Authenticity 15

3.6 Navigating the Winds of Change 16

Chapter 4: The Song of Resilience - Overcoming Fear and Resistance 17

Resistance to change can be a major obstacle in your journey toward better hearing. Uncover the song of resilience within you, and learn to face your fears and doubts to embrace the transformative power of self-improvement.

> 4.1 The Melody of Courage 17
> 4.2 The Harmonies of Hope 17
> 4.3 The Rhythm of Adaptability 18
> 4.4 The Chorus of Support 18
> 4.5 The Bridge of Perseverance 18
> 4.6 The Crescendo of Empowerment 19

Chapter 5: The Rhythm of Change - Finding Motivation to Take Action 20

Motivation is the driving force behind any significant change in life. Explore the rhythm of change and learn to tap into your own unique sources of motivation, which will propel you toward a better understanding of your hearing health.

> 5.1 The Beat of Inspiration 20
> 5.2 The Tempo of Goal Setting 20
> 5.3 The Dynamics of Self-Belief 21
> 5.4 The Harmony of Balance 21
> 5.5 The Syncopation of Accountability 21
> 5.6 The Crescendo of Progress 22

Chapter 6: The Harmony of Support - Building a Network of Understanding 23

A network of support is vital when facing any challenge in life. Learn how to create a harmony of understanding among your friends, family, and healthcare professionals who can assist you on your journey.

    6.1 The Chords of Connection 23

    6.2 The Ensemble of Professionals 24

    6.3 The Melody of Shared Experience 24

    6.4 The Refrain of Advocacy 24

    6.5 The Bridge of Reciprocity 25

    6.6 The Crescendo of Resilience 25

Chapter 7: The Crescendo of Transformation - Taking Charge of Your Hearing Health 27

As you continue to embrace change and rediscover your world of sound, you'll experience a crescendo of transformation. Learn how to take charge of your hearing health and experience the joy and fulfillment that comes from being an active participant in the symphony of life.

    7.1 The Overture of Awareness 27

    7.2 The Symphony of Action 27

    7.3 The Coda of Consistency 28

    7.4 The Rondo of Adaptation 28

    7.5 The Canon of Self-Advocacy 28

    7.6 The Finale of Empowerment 29

Conclusion: The Overture to a New Beginning 30

Introduction

Imagine life as a symphony, a beautiful blend of sounds and melodies that create a unique, immersive experience. For some, however, certain notes and harmonies may fade or be altogether absent, leaving a sense of incompleteness in the music of life. Hearing loss is a challenge that affects many, but finding the motivation and courage to face it head-on can make all the difference in rediscovering the richness of the world around you.

In the spirit of C. Rogers' empathetic and compassionate approach, this book is meant to be a gentle yet powerful exploration of self-discovery, acceptance, and change for those who are experiencing hearing loss. Through meaningful metaphors and inspiring examples, we aim to awaken your motivation and empower you to take charge of your health and well-being.

Chapter 1:
The Silent Garden - Acknowledging Your Hearing Loss

The first step in any journey of change begins with acknowledging the reality of your situation. Just as the gardener must recognize the state of their garden to nurture it back to life, you too must come to terms with the reality of your hearing loss. In this chapter, we'll explore the process of acknowledging your hearing loss and how it can serve as a catalyst for positive change.

1.1 The Beauty in Silence

In the quiet moments of life, we often find solace and reflection. The silent garden, with its fading flowers and quiet corners, can be a place of introspection, allowing you to come to terms with your hearing loss. It is in these moments of stillness that we find the opportunity to truly listen to our inner voice and begin to understand the changes that have occurred in our lives. Embracing the silence can be the first step toward acknowledging your hearing loss and finding the motivation to seek help.

1.2 The Fading Notes

As you walk through the silent garden, you may notice that certain notes, once vibrant and resonant, have begun to fade away. This is a metaphor for the gradual nature of hearing loss, which often progresses slowly over time. By recognizing these fading notes and acknowledging their absence, you are taking an important step in understanding the impact of your hearing loss on your life.

1.3 The Seeds of Change

In every garden, there lies the potential for renewal and growth. As you acknowledge your hearing loss, you are planting the seeds of change that will eventually blossom into a renewed sense of self and an improved quality of life. By admitting the reality of your situation, you are laying the groundwork for personal growth and paving the way for positive change.

1.4 Cultivating Self-Compassion

Acknowledging your hearing loss can be an emotional and difficult experience, but it is essential to approach this process with self-compassion. Treat yourself with kindness, understanding, and patience, as you would a friend facing a similar challenge. By extending this compassion to yourself, you create a nurturing environment that will allow the seeds of change to take root and grow.

1.5 The Power of Vulnerability

Admitting to yourself and others that you are experiencing hearing loss requires a great deal of vulnerability. By opening yourself up to this vulnerability, you are inviting support and understanding from those around you. This can be a powerful catalyst for change, as it fosters a sense of connection and empathy that can help propel you forward on your journey.

1.6 Turning the Soil

Once you have acknowledged your hearing loss, it is time to turn the soil and prepare for the next steps in your journey. This may involve seeking professional help, researching treatment options, or connecting with others who share your experience. As you turn the soil, you are creating a fertile environment for change, one that is rich with possibility and opportunity.

In conclusion, acknowledging your hearing loss is the first and most crucial step in your journey toward better hearing. Like the gardener who tends to the silent garden, you must recognize the reality of your situation and embrace the potential for growth and renewal. By doing so, you are planting the seeds of change that will ultimately lead to a richer, more fulfilling life, filled with the vibrant sounds of the world around you.

Chapter 2:
The Echo of Self-Acceptance - Embracing Your Reality

Self-acceptance is a powerful and transformative force that can propel you forward on your journey toward better hearing. In this chapter, we will explore the importance of self-acceptance, how to cultivate it, and the impact it can have on your life as you embrace your reality and move forward.

2.1 The Sound of Acceptance

Imagine standing in a canyon and shouting your truth into the void. The echoes of your voice reverberate, creating a powerful affirmation of self-acceptance. This metaphor illustrates the significance of embracing your reality and accepting your hearing loss. As you accept your situation, you create an echo of self-affirmation that grows stronger, resonating within you and empowering your journey toward better hearing.

2.2 The Layers of Self-Acceptance

Self-acceptance is a multifaceted concept, consisting of several layers. It involves acknowledging your hearing loss, embracing your imperfections, and recognizing your inherent worth. By peeling back these layers and cultivating self-acceptance, you create a strong foundation for personal growth and change.

2.3 The Mirror of Self-Reflection

The journey toward self-acceptance often begins with self-reflection. Like gazing into a mirror, self-reflection allows you to see yourself clearly and without judgment. By taking an honest and compassionate look at yourself, you can begin to accept your hearing loss and understand its impact on your life. This process helps you develop a sense of empathy and understanding toward yourself, making it easier to accept your reality.

2.4 The Warmth of Self-Compassion

Self-compassion is an essential component of self-acceptance. By treating yourself with kindness, patience, and understanding, you create a nurturing environment that fosters self-acceptance. Remember that self-compassion is not about denying your hearing loss or minimizing its impact; it's about embracing your reality with love and support.

2.5 The Strength of Vulnerability

As you work toward self-acceptance, you may encounter feelings of vulnerability. Embrace this vulnerability and recognize it as a source of strength, rather than weakness. By allowing yourself to be open and honest about your hearing loss, you are taking a courageous step toward self-acceptance and personal growth.

2.6 The Ripple Effect of Acceptance

Self-acceptance has a powerful ripple effect, extending beyond yourself and into your relationships and interactions with others. By embracing your reality and accepting your hearing loss, you cultivate an atmosphere of openness and honesty, which can lead to deeper connections with friends, family, and loved ones. This ripple effect can also inspire others to practice self-acceptance and cultivate empathy for those around them.

In conclusion, the echo of self-acceptance is a crucial aspect of your journey toward better hearing. By cultivating self-acceptance, you are creating a powerful foundation for personal growth and change. Embrace your reality, and allow the echoes of self-acceptance to reverberate through your life, inspiring and empowering you as you take charge of your hearing health and reconnect with the world of sound.

Chapter 3:
The Whispering Wind - Listening to Your Inner Voice

Your inner voice can serve as a guiding force on your journey toward better hearing. Often subtle and soft like a whispering wind, it can easily be drowned out by the noise of self-doubt, fear, or external influences. In this chapter, we'll explore how to listen to your inner voice, trust your intuition, and use it to make decisions that align with your goals and values.

3.1 The Gentle Breeze of Intuition

Intuition is a powerful, innate force that can guide you through life's challenges, including the journey to better hearing. Like a gentle breeze that carries whispers of wisdom, your intuition can provide insights and guidance when you take the time to listen and tune in to its subtle messages.

3.2 Clearing the Mental Clutter

To effectively listen to your inner voice, it's essential to clear the mental clutter that can often drown it out. This may involve practicing mindfulness, meditation, or journaling to quiet the noise of everyday life and create space for your intuition to be heard.

3.3 Trusting Your Inner Guidance

Learning to trust your inner voice is a crucial aspect of embracing your intuition. As you begin to pay attention to the whispering wind of your inner guidance, you'll discover that it often leads you toward choices that align with your values and goals. Trusting your intuition requires a leap of faith, but as you do so, you'll find that it becomes a reliable and empowering force in your life.

3.4 Overcoming Self-Doubt

Self-doubt can be a significant barrier to listening to and trusting your inner voice. By acknowledging and confronting these doubts, you can begin to overcome them and create space for your intuition to thrive. Remind yourself of your strengths, accomplishments, and inherent worth, and trust that your inner voice is guiding you toward a path of self-improvement and growth.

3.5 The Power of Authenticity

Authenticity is closely tied to the ability to listen to and trust your inner voice. By embracing your true self and honoring your feelings and experiences, you create an environment where your intuition can flourish. As you cultivate authenticity, you'll find that your inner voice becomes a more potent and reliable source of guidance.

3.6 Navigating the Winds of Change

As you embark on your journey toward better hearing, your inner voice can serve as a compass, helping you navigate the winds of change. By tuning in to your intuition and trusting its guidance, you'll be better equipped to make decisions that lead to a more fulfilling and healthy life.

In conclusion, the whispering wind of your inner voice is a powerful ally in your quest for better hearing. By learning to listen to, trust, and embrace your intuition, you'll find that it becomes a guiding force in your life, leading you toward self-improvement and a deeper connection with the world of sound. Remember that your inner voice is always there, whispering its wisdom like a gentle breeze. All you need to do is listen.

Chapter 4:
The Song of Resilience - Overcoming Fear and Resistance

The journey toward better hearing can be fraught with fear and resistance. Change can be challenging, and the unknown can evoke feelings of anxiety and trepidation. In this chapter, we'll explore the song of resilience, the powerful melody that can help you face your fears, overcome resistance, and embrace the transformative power of self-improvement.

4.1 The Melody of Courage

Resilience is often born from courage. By facing your fears and embracing the unknown, you create a powerful melody that resonates within your soul. This melody of courage can help you overcome obstacles, navigate change, and persevere in your quest for better hearing.

4.2 The Harmonies of Hope

Hope is a vital component of resilience. By focusing on the positive aspects of your journey and maintaining an optimistic outlook, you can create harmonies of hope that complement the melody of courage. These harmonies can serve as a reminder that even in the face of adversity, there is always the possibility of growth, change, and improvement.

4.3 The Rhythm of Adaptability

Resilience requires adaptability, the ability to adjust to new circumstances and embrace change with grace. By developing a rhythm of adaptability, you can navigate the ups and downs of your journey and continue to move forward, even when faced with setbacks or challenges.

4.4 The Chorus of Support

A strong support system is crucial in building resilience. By surrounding yourself with friends, family, and professionals who understand your journey, you create a chorus of support that can bolster your courage and help you overcome fear and resistance. This chorus can provide encouragement, advice, and a listening ear when you need it most.

4.5 The Bridge of Perseverance

Perseverance is the bridge that connects fear and resistance to growth and transformation. By cultivating a sense of determination and persistence, you can cross this bridge and continue on your path toward better hearing. Recognize that setbacks are a natural part of any journey, and use them as an opportunity to learn and grow.

4.6 The Crescendo of Empowerment

As you develop resilience, you'll experience a crescendo of empowerment. This newfound sense of strength and self-reliance can provide the motivation and energy needed to tackle the challenges of your journey and embrace the transformative power of change.

In conclusion, the song of resilience is a powerful anthem that can help you face your fears, overcome resistance, and move forward on your journey toward better hearing. By cultivating courage, hope, adaptability, and perseverance, you can create a symphony of strength that will guide you through the challenges and opportunities that lie ahead. Remember that the song of resilience is always within you, ready to be sung whenever you need a reminder of your inner strength and the transformative power of change.

Chapter 5:
The Rhythm of Change - Finding Motivation to Take Action

Motivation is the driving force that propels us toward change and self-improvement. In this chapter, we'll explore the rhythm of change and how you can find the motivation to take action, embrace your hearing loss journey, and transform your life for the better.

5.1 The Beat of Inspiration

Inspiration can provide the spark needed to ignite your motivation. Reflect on your reasons for seeking better hearing, whether it's to strengthen relationships, enhance your career, or simply improve your overall quality of life. By connecting with these sources of inspiration, you can tap into the beat that drives you to take action.

5.2 The Tempo of Goal Setting

Setting realistic and achievable goals can help you maintain motivation and focus on your journey toward better hearing. Break down your overarching

Chapter 6:
The Harmony of Support - Building a Network of Understanding

The journey toward better hearing can be challenging, but you don't have to face it alone. A network of understanding and support can provide the harmony needed to navigate the ups and downs of this transformative path. In this chapter, we'll explore how to build a strong support system and the invaluable role it plays in your journey to improved hearing.

6.1 The Chords of Connection

Connection is at the heart of any support network. Begin by reaching out to friends, family, and loved ones, sharing your experiences and feelings about your hearing loss journey. By opening up and fostering these chords of connection, you create a foundation of understanding and empathy upon which your support network can be built.

6.2 The Ensemble of Professionals

In addition to your personal connections, it's essential to include professionals in your support network. Audiologists, hearing healthcare providers, and therapists can provide expert guidance, advice, and resources to help you navigate your journey. Assemble your ensemble of professionals to ensure you have a well-rounded and knowledgeable team supporting you every step of the way.

6.3 The Melody of Shared Experience

Support groups can offer a unique sense of understanding and camaraderie, as they are often comprised of individuals who share similar experiences and challenges. By joining a support group, either in person or online, you can tap into the melody of shared experience, providing encouragement, insights, and the reassurance that you're not alone in your journey.

6.4 The Refrain of Advocacy

Empowering yourself through education and advocacy is a crucial aspect of building a strong support network. By learning about hearing loss and advocating for your needs, you can create a supportive environment that fosters understanding and empathy among those around you. This refrain of advocacy can be a powerful tool for building and maintaining your support network.

6.5 The Bridge of Reciprocity

As you build your support network, remember the importance of reciprocity. Offering support and understanding to others in your network not only strengthens your connections but also reinforces your sense of self-worth and purpose. By being there for others, you'll find that the harmony of support becomes even more powerful and meaningful.

6.6 The Crescendo of Resilience

A strong support network can create a crescendo of resilience, bolstering your ability to face challenges and overcome obstacles on your journey to better hearing. By surrounding yourself with understanding, empathy, and encouragement, you'll be better equipped to navigate the ups and downs of your journey and emerge stronger and more resilient than ever.

In conclusion, the harmony of support is a vital aspect of your journey toward better hearing. By building a network of understanding that includes personal connections, professionals, support groups, and a focus on advocacy and reciprocity, you can create a powerful and enduring support system that will see you through the challenges and triumphs of your transformative journey. Embrace the harmony of support, and let its comforting notes guide and uplift you as you forge ahead on your path to improved hearing.

Chapter 7:
The Crescendo of Transformation - Taking Charge of Your Hearing Health

As you embark on your journey toward better hearing, you will experience a crescendo of transformation, marked by growth, change, and self-discovery. In this final chapter, we'll explore how to take charge of your hearing health and embrace the transformative power of self-improvement.

7.1 The Overture of Awareness

Your journey begins with awareness—recognizing your hearing loss and the impact it has on your life. This overture of awareness is the starting point from which you can begin to take charge of your hearing health and set the stage for the transformative process that lies ahead.

7.2 The Symphony of Action

With awareness comes the opportunity to take action. By seeking professional help, exploring treatment options, and following a personalized care plan, you can orchestrate a symphony of action that leads to improved hearing and a better quality of life.

7.3 The Coda of Consistency

Consistency is key to taking charge of your hearing health. By adhering to your care plan, practicing good hearing health habits, and attending regular follow-up appointments, you can maintain a coda of consistency that will support your ongoing transformation.

7.4 The Rondo of Adaptation

As you progress on your journey, you will encounter new challenges and opportunities for growth. Embrace the rondo of adaptation by being open to change, adjusting your approach as needed, and continually learning from your experiences.

7.5 The Canon of Self-Advocacy

Taking charge of your hearing health also involves becoming an advocate for yourself. By educating yourself about hearing loss, communicating your needs, and seeking accommodations when necessary, you can create a canon of self-advocacy that empowers you to take control of your life and your hearing journey.

7.6 The Finale of Empowerment

As you navigate the crescendo of transformation, you will ultimately reach a finale of empowerment. This newfound sense of strength, self-reliance, and confidence will enable you to face challenges with resilience, celebrate your successes, and continue to grow and evolve on your journey to better hearing.

In conclusion, the crescendo of transformation is the culmination of your journey toward taking charge of your hearing health. By cultivating awareness, taking action, maintaining consistency, adapting to change, advocating for yourself, and ultimately embracing empowerment, you can unlock the full potential of your hearing journey and experience the life-changing benefits of better hearing. As the final notes of your transformative symphony ring out, remember that you have the power to shape your own destiny and create a life filled with harmony, connection, and fulfillment.

Conclusion:
The Overture to a New Beginning

Your journey toward better hearing is an ongoing process of self-discovery, acceptance, and change. This book serves as an overture to a new beginning, one in which you can experience the richness and beauty of the world around you. May the symphony of life play on, inspiring you to embrace the challenges and opportunities that lie ahead.

With compassion, empathy, and understanding, we hope this book will serve as a beacon of hope, guiding you toward the path of self-improvement and reconnection with the world of sound. Remember, the music of life is waiting for you. All you need to do is listen.

www.ingramcontent.com/pod-product-compliance
Lightning Source LLC
Chambersburg PA
CBHW040301220526
45473CB00002B/553